# Weight-Loss Failure Is NOT Your Fault!

*Learn the ONLY True Path to Permanent Success*

**By David D. Erickson**

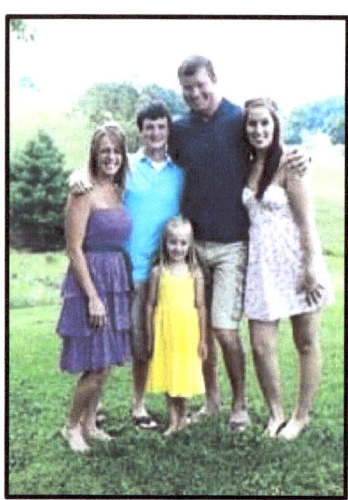

The Erickson family: Jenny, Taylor, Elle, Dave and Chelsie

**We all live to be our best,** for ourselves, and for those we Love. Living in peace, balance, and joy is not only our mission, but our responsibility as parents and mature adults. Providing for our families is not just going to work to pay the bills and take our kids to Disney World®, but to be a role model of happiness and good health in a world of stress and dysfunction. Families are most often broken because of the parents' feelings of being out of control and an inner dislike of themselves, which causes defensiveness, judgment, and perpetual fighting. Our children are growing
up adopting our most commonly used coping tool—overeating. We parents are often oblivious to, or choose to ignore, how our behavior is being
learned and locked-in as powerful habits our children will struggle with as adults!

Now is YOUR time to stop the insanity of living your life one more day disliking yourself, passing on habits, and going on another "diet" that will only be another blow to your self-image.

In these pages you will find the ONLY path to permanent weight-loss fully described and laid out for you to follow – a path that leads to freedom, peace, balance, and a new life! And at the end of the book, Dave will be there to help you take this path and succeed!

# Contents

4

We've all heard the dismal statistics; 90% of diets fail. Gyms and Fitness Centers are packed in January and empty by March. We are getting fatter—now 60% of Americas are overweight despite the literally thousands of diet books and programs available. And surveys show that half of those who are overweight are currently trying to lose weight.

> Weight-loss isn't about numbers
> and statistics.
> It's about individuals and
> how they feel about themselves.

Consumers spend more than $35 Billion on weight-loss products and programs every year. This figure includes sales of books, videos, tapes, low-calorie foods and drinks, sugar substitutes, meal replacements, prescription drugs, over-the-counter drugs, dietary supplements, medical treatments, commercial weight-loss chains, and other products or services related to weight-loss or weight maintenance. Despite this massive spending and desire for weight-loss, the vast majority of people who set out with good intentions of losing weight end up failing. But weight-loss failure, as I will show you, is not your fault!

How you feel about yourself affects everything that you value in your life. Quickly make a mental list of the four most important things in your life. Most would list kids, spouse, family and career. When you feel good about yourself you are a more patient and loving parent. When you feel good about yourself you are a more forgiving and understanding spouse. When you feel good about yourself you are a more helpful and considerate brother, sister, son or daughter. When you feel good about yourself you are a more productive and positive team player at work.

Imagine the result of living the next 5, 10, 20 or more years of YOUR life feeling really good about yourself, and the massive positive results it could allow you to produce in your life!

**Weight loss is not about vanity, it's about your life!**

## ABOUT THE AUTHOR

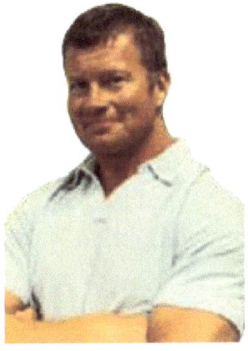

In 1997, I was unemployed with an MBA, looking for what I wanted to do with my life. Two years earlier I had ended a short career going from stock boy to assistant store manager for Wal-Mart and went to grad school to get my MBA. After proudly graduating with a 4.0 GPA, I decided after looking for a job for a few months that what I really wanted was to own my own business—but it had to be something I loved.

That was a simple decision; I loved working out and helping people. I decided to take my American Council on Exercise (ACE) Personal Trainer certification and my MBA, and open a gym to help people improve their lives through exercise and weight-loss! Everything fell into place, including a $10,000 gift from a great aunt who had just passed away and a newly-built vacant building for lease in a small town with no fitness center. In the fall of 1997, I opened Fit4Life Fitness Center "*Fitness for All Ages and Abilities*" in Sparta, Wisconsin. My small gym began to grow and in just 3 years I moved to a larger building.

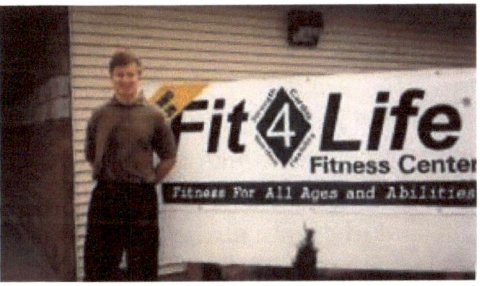

Today, I own two gyms and now I train other trainers to help people lose weight and get fit. For the first ten years, I trained and assisted hundreds of people with their weight-loss and fitness goals. I experienced over and over again how difficult it is for people who decide to lose weight to actually do it!

I could teach a person all the skills they needed to succeed, but most of the time I couldn't motivate them to fully follow through to get the results they came to me for. I had lots of short-term success with clients, but not a lot of long-term success.

Why do human beings make good intentions
for really good reasons
and then fail to follow-through time after time?!

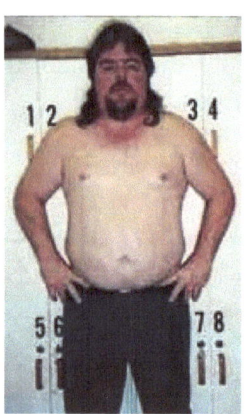 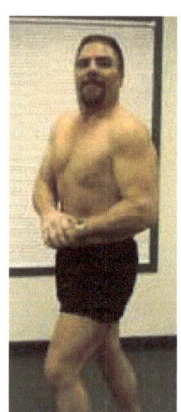 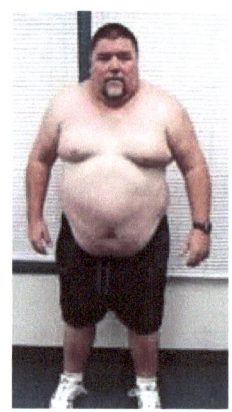

One of my clients: Richard, a truck driver, lost over 100 pounds, but a few years later gained it all back and then some! I remember lying in bed thinking I would eventually have everyone in the area join the gym, fail to reach their goal, quit the gym, and I'd eventually be out of business! Over the years, I just accepted this as a "fact of life". It wasn't until I started training other trainers to successfully help their clients lose weight that I recognized the need to find a better answer than "that's just the way it is." I had also just turned 40, and was starting to ask myself a very motivat-

ing question: *"What am I going to do with the rest of my life?"*
Combine these two powerful forces to find answers and I
was a man on a mission!

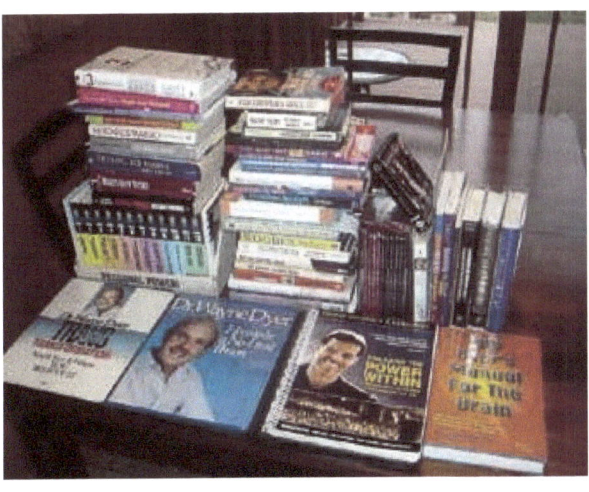

Over two years, I read dozens of books on everything I could
get my hands on including topics like self-hypnosis,
visualization, Neuro-Linguistic Programming (NLP),
personal change and self-improvement. I even attended a 4-
day live seminar with Tony Robbins in which I walked across
12-feet of burning coals!

I listened to cassette tapes and CDs from these authors in
my car everywhere I drove. I even recorded this stuff on my
iPod and took books with me when we went on vacations.
You could say I went bonkers - just ask my wife! I couldn't get
enough because I was finding the answers! I was having one
"aha!" discovery and distinction after another, making
everything make sense! *"Man, I just gotta share this stuff with
other people!"* I kept telling myself.

## DRIVING DOWN THE WRONG ROAD

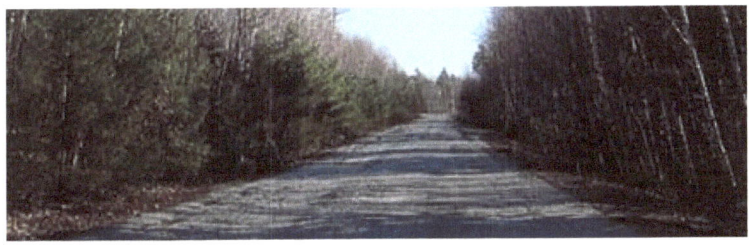

Ever driven down the wrong road? Feels like crap once you discover you've just spent the last 15 minutes driving 10 miles the wrong way! Imagine what it would feel like driving down the wrong road for 15 days, 61 days or 169 days? How many days did your last weight-loss program last? Now imagine driving down the wrong road for 169 days, not arriving at the destination you wanted and then a few months or a year later, maybe on January 1st, deciding to go to the same destination named "what-I'd-like-to-weigh" and driving down the same darn road! This is what everyone is doing! Why? Everyone thinks there's only one road!

## There IS Another Road!

The road of "failed-good-intentions" is the road of using willpower to reach the destination. We humans believe the yellow brick road to personal change is to use our will or resolve, self-discipline, or character to make the change. We decide consciously to lose weight, quit smoking, stop procrastination, stop or start whatever, and we use our conscious will to force ourselves to do the opposite of what our inner feelings compel us to do. The big problem with this approach is we overwhelmingly underestimate the power of our inner feelings powered by our subconscious brain and, when they eventually win out over our willpower, we believe the reason we failed was because of our personal lack of resolve, self-discipline or character. *This is a huge blow to one's self-esteem and confidence.* The exciting truth

I discovered and will share with you in this book is that it's not your fault! Yes, let me repeat that. It's _not_ _YOUR fault_! Everyone's brain is designed in a way that makes the willpower road to personal change horribly frustrating, painful and ineffective!

The road of "successful change" is the road of changing your inner feelings so that you want to do what you consciously would like to do. We all know people who want to and like to exercise and eat healthy. They love it. They don't need to use their willpower to get themselves to go to the gym or to eat a salad for lunch. That's their inner feeling, which compels them automatically.

Don't you wish I could just wave my magic wand over your head and "presto" your inner desires would fall in line with what you wanted to do! I attended a seminar on weight-loss hypnosis and everyone in the audience had given up on his or her own ability to lose weight. They all were there for the same reason. They each paid $59 in hopes that hypnosis would be their "magic wand" to change them on the inside so they could gain control of their overeating and lazy desires.

In this book, I will teach you how to get on the _only_ road of successful change. It's not remotely as difficult as you might think to change your inner desires. In fact, most of what I will be teaching you, you already do—you're just not aware and in charge of it yet! I am extremely excited for you and this opportunity we have to REALLY help you accomplish the long-term success you deserve! I promise to give you my best! What I'm going to teach you all starts with some understanding.......

## WHY WE WANT TO BE THIN

In our society it's no secret that we judge people by their appearance. Overweight people are treated differently and certain assumptions are attached to them, such as "Overweight people are lazy or lack self-discipline." No one wants to be labeled or judged negatively. So this, along with the fact that we subconsciously assume thin people to be more attractive, hardworking, intelligent and successful, is the reason for our strong desire to be thin.

## WHY WE LOVE FOOD

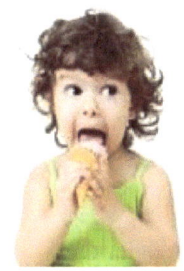

We are all mentally wired to enjoy food for obvious survival reasons. But we're specifically wired to enjoy high carbohydrate and high fat food. This makes sense because fat contains the most calories per gram and carbohydrates are our body's preferred fuel source. Furthermore, there's a strong conditioning effect that takes place when we give our children birthday cake, candy, cookies, high-sugar beverages, chips, etc., during fun times like birthday parties, as rewards for good behavior, and as a way to make a child feel better after a physical injury or hurt feelings.

Our brains become powerfully conditioned
to associate high fat/high carb foods
with higher levels of pleasure and feeling loved.

So no wonder we have a strong pull toward high fat/carb foods; they create powerful feelings of pleasure, both physically and psychologically. This explains why people who don't feel satisfied and happy with their life easily turn to high carb/fat food to gain this needed feeling. The human brain must feel good. It's designed to move you

13

away from pain and toward pleasure automatically. Bad feelings stimulate a person to take some action to get back to feeling good. Just open up the newspaper and you'll see my point illustrated in sad stories of people who did dumb or destructive things to get back to feeling good. This design of our brains is so powerful, we'll do things we know are destructive long- term, just to avoid pain and/or get pleasure in the short- term. The father who kidnaps his son after losing custody is a perfect example of a man who needed to get out of the immediate pain of not seeing his son. But long-term the man goes to prison, loses his son and makes his pain even worse!

The greater the pain, the more a person is guided by their subconscious needs, and the less they are guided by their conscious thinking, causing them to do things for short-term gain despite certain massive long-term loss.

Overeaters exhibit this very same natural behavior. They have issues or circumstances in their life making them feel "pain" (disappointed, depressed, overwhelmed, frustrated, bored, angry, rejected, nervous, etc.) and are sub-consciously driven to overeat to eliminate the painful feelings by experiencing the highly pleasurable feeling of enjoying the taste of the high fat/carb food and indulging in this positive feeling until physically satisfied (full). However, after they've gained this short-term pleasure, they feel bad about themselves from their inability to control their eating which then reduces their self-esteem and willpower. This cycle will repeat itself until the person finds or creates other things in their life that makes them feel satisfied and happy, or they eliminate or learn to live with the things that are giving them negative feelings.

## THE DILEMMA

Because of our strong natural desire to eat high fat and carb foods, we want to keep eating and enjoying these foods in unrestricted quantities but also have the pleasures that come from possessing an attractive body. "Eat whatever you want and still lose weight!" type of ads, are by far the most appealing and successful. Weight-loss programs that allow pleasure eating and low amounts of physical effort are very alluring to us humans who often want opposing things. It's similar to a husband being drawn to having a girlfriend and still wanting to stay happily married. From our natural desire to "have our cake and eat it too", many people have developed mentalities that ensure weight-loss failure.

## "TAKE A PILL" MENTALITY

The way we "fix" other health problems in our life has con-ditioned us to believe there must also be a similar way to

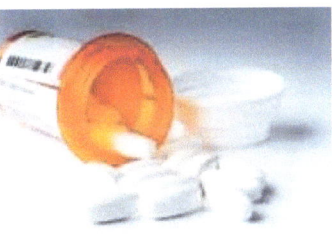

"fix" our overweight problem. If we have a health problem, most of the time we are sent home with a prescription for a bottle of pills which, if we take them over time, solves our health problem. So we begin to believe that if we are sick or have a physical problem, taking a pill is often the answer to getting better. The allure of this method of solving our physical problems is mesmerizing! What could be easier than just taking a few tiny pills to solve your problem? Results with little effort is highly attractive.

## GAMBLER'S MENTALITY

When you gamble, you do the same thing over and over with the expectation of a potential different outcome. You push the button on the slot machine over and over with the expectation of winning if you just keep pushing the button. People wanting to lose weight often take this same approach. If they just keep trying, eventually, they'll lose the weight. They start a diet and fail. After a certain time period, they start another diet and fail. Some join a gym and end up not going. After 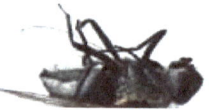 a certain period of time, they rejoin the gym and quit going again. After a period of time, they rejoin a different gym, but after time fail again. Most people keep repeating the same pattern over and over again. It's like a fly bouncing against a closed window trying to get outside. The fly keeps doing the same thing: flying into the glass over and over until eventually you find him legs up and dead on the window sill! The only way the fly will get outside, or the dieter will be successful, is if he learns from his failed attempts and takes a new approach each time, until he or she finds a path to success!

## THE HIGH COST OF FAILURE

When one fails to lose weight, much more is lost than just the money spent on the products or services. When a person fails at weight-loss, they lose their precious confidence and self-esteem. Failing at weight-loss, I would argue, is more psychologically damaging to a person than failing at other intentions because of the emotions attached to the deep desire of living in an attractive body. This is why people are motivated to keep trying to lose weight even after failing many times! When one fails at weight-loss, their self-definition often becomes: "*I'm unattractive and I'm a failure too.*" When a person dislikes themselves, many self-defeating beliefs and behaviors can become a part of the person's life, including:

- Covering up their feelings about themselves & their life with additional eating, drinking or drugs.

16

- Being drawn to criticize others constantly including loved ones and friends in order to compensate and feel better about themselves.

- Becoming depressed, less motivated and more confrontational at work, causing reprimands, warnings, or firing.

- Becoming less motivated at home, causing more arguments and relationship problems.

- Becoming more needy of acceptance and approval from others to feel good about themselves, making them a slave to what others think.

- Becoming highly sensitive to failure, and fearing to try anything outside of what is comfortable, resulting in a life that doesn't improve or grow.

- Becoming highly sensitive to any criticism, causing people to avoid them.

- Believing they have no control over how they feel because of the "unfair world", resulting in an attitude of "life is crap" which causes them to interpret many things that happen in their life as negative or against them. This forces them to find some way to overcome this painful feeling—the easiest and most common method is the enjoyment of high carb or fat foods.

A 2009 study in the Archives of General Psychiatry found that antidepressant drug use increased 75% from 1996 to 2005, from about 6% of the population in 1996 to over 10% in 2005. This number is now closer to 15% (2013).

It's easy to make the correlation between the millions of

people wanting deeply to lose weight and to feel attractive and the rising use of antidepressants. Furthermore, it's not a person's actual weight, but a person's *perceived* dissatisfaction with their weight that is the determining factor. You can be a healthy weight but still be depressed because you think you would be more attractive if you weighed less.

No question, the cost of trying to lose weight and failing is very high!

## YOU MUST FEEL GREAT TO LOSE WEIGHT

Most people have this backwards. They believe they need to lose weight before they can feel good about themselves. This is natural, but is the major reason why people fail to lose weight. How you feel emotionally determines your level of motivation. When faced with an eating decision between a frozen pizza or taking time to cook-up something healthy, you must be in positive state of mind. If you're feeling depressed, hurt, frustrated or overwhelmed, which option do you think you will choose?

Think about it, when you're feeling excited and confident, don't you feel like doing things you would never feel like doing when you feel tired and frustrated?

Most people believe that other people and the environment control how we feel, but in reality, how we choose to perceive things determines the emotions we choose to experience. One person can perceive hosting Thanksgiving dinner as a "burden" and be stressed out about every detail. Another person can perceive hosting any family event as a "blessing" by focusing on the people coming and the wonderful fellowship of such an event.

Gaining control of your emotions is essential to gaining control of what you do.

One person gets fired and goes into depression and can't motivate himself to send out resumes, make calls or pursue a new job; he feels too down. His colleague decides to give the firing a new meaning of opportunity; she decides to feel good about this highly motivating opportunity to finally get off her butt and find a better job! With her inner enthusiasm, she gets hired at a better paying job in less than 3 months!

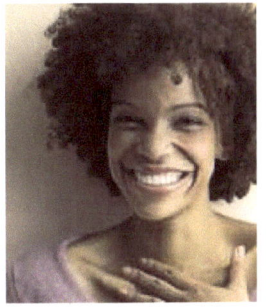

Every event in your life that makes you feel
a negative emotion
can be looked at differently to create
a positive emotion.

When trying to lose weight, most people are like the person who feels down about getting fired, goes out and interviews poorly, and fails! People who have failed at weight-loss time and time again feel down about their ability to lose weight, and thus put forth a weak effort the next time they attempt to lose weight and thus fail again. This is called the "**Cycle of Failure**".

This is why it is SO important to
hammer home the message
that your past weight-loss failures were
NOT YOUR FAULT!

You can't lose weight if you feel down about yourself!

Ask yourself which of the following charts of
emotional states
best describes YOUR daily life

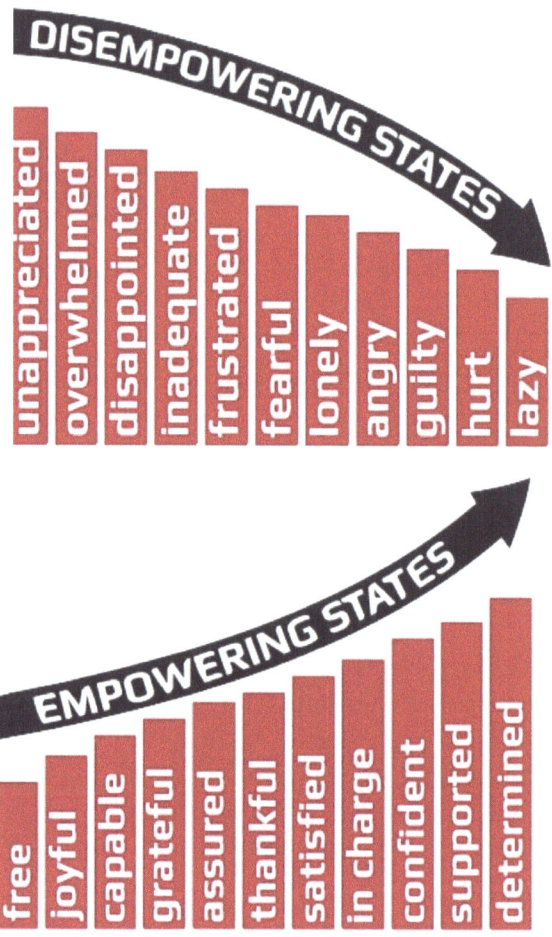

If how you feel most often is described better in the top chart than in the bottom, you're going to struggle with weight-loss no matter how much you know about it. You can read a dozen books on weight-loss skills and know as much as I do about how to eat and exercise correctly to produce fat loss, but if you're held captive to the emotions described in the left column, when it comes time to decide "frozen pizza or veggies?", you'll choose frozen pizza more than you choose veggies!

Gaining the skills to put yourself into your most resourceful, empowering states and leave behind your disempowering states is essential for weight-loss success!

## WHY PEOPLE FAIL TO LOSE WEIGHT

When a person fails at a good intention, they tend to believe that they must not possess enough "willpower". Willpower is believed to be a personal trait by many—some genetic or learned attribute that one either has or doesn't have. But the truth of the matter is that everyone has willpower. Let me give you an example. Parents of a young teenager thought he lacked willpower because he failed in school and was lazy a round the home. However, this same young man had the "willpower" to find a way to a rock concert 100 miles away with only $5 in his pocket! Because the teenager really, re- ally wanted to go to the concert, he did whatever it took to get there.

Willpower or motivation to do something comes from having a strong emotional reason to do it. For the teenager, the reason his willpower was off the charts to get to the rock concert was because a certain girl he's crazy about said she was going and hinted she'd hang out with him if he went!

The reason people fail to lose weight is because their reasons or "whys" are not motivating enough. Any difficult personal change has to be motivated by powerful "whys" that make changing a must. It's never usually a matter of ability; it's a matter of motivation. To prove my point, if I were to kidnap your kids, and not until you lost 20 pounds would they be returned to you safely, would you be able to lose the weight?

21

*out ice cream before bed anymore!*" or "*To hell with all this exercise!*" I would bet not. You'd do whatever it took to lose the 20 pounds. Failure would not be an option because you'd have a very powerful "why". Losing 20 pounds would become a must!

Willpower is generated from how emotionally powerful your reasons are to accomplish your goal.

## WEAK "WHYS" ARE NATURAL

Have you ever put your whole heart into something and failed? Hurt really bad didn't it? The more of ourselves we invest into anything, the added risk we take of getting hurt. This fear of failure then causes most people to approach weight-loss with half-hearted efforts and a lack of sufficient focus and priority. Furthermore, the allure and myth of easy weight-loss causes most folks to believe that weight-loss can be accomplished with less effort than it actually takes. We are inundated with commercials and advertising that teach us to believe weight-loss is possible with minimal effort. Many people still believe there is a "secret" exercise or "secret" eating method or program that when they find it, will give them the correct path to easy weight-loss. These thoughts are often reinforced by thinner friends who find exercise to be an enjoyable part of their life and eat high-calorie foods at weekend parties or restaurants. It's easy to believe this is how their thinner friends always eat and still stay fit—they must have found the "secret". Such beliefs don't necessitate a strong resolve or the need to find strong "whys".

Perhaps the strongest reason for weak "whys" is the assumption that if an intention is for a good reason, then the motivation to do it should be automatic. When what we've decided to do will drastically improve our lives, or even save our life, it just makes sense. There'd be something wrong with us if we didn't! But this is not the case. Many people with very good intentions to quit smoking, lose weight or spend more time with the kids find themselves back smok- ing, overeating and ignoring their kids! This widely held belief that a good intention itself should be enough of a "why" to motivate follow-through causes a person who fails to believe there must be something wrong with them. The man who sets the good intention to spend more time with his kids, and fails, begins to believe he's not a good parent and feels less of himself.

Powerful "whys" - I MUST
= strong willpower
= goal is my priority & focus

Weak "whys" - I SHOULD
= weak motivation
= goal is not my priority or focus

## HOW TO FIND & CREATE YOUR POWERFUL "WHYS"

**Everything that you do is motivated by two and only two forces:**
### 1. Avoiding pain
### 2. Gaining pleasure
**All human behavior is motivated by one or both of these forces.**

Understanding how the twin forces of Pain and Pleasure are compelling you to do things you'd like to change helps you to understand how to use these forces to compel yourself to do what you really want. Procrastination, for example, occurs when the pain of doing something is greater than the pain of not doing it, so you naturally are compelled to avoid the pain by putting it off. Only until a deadline with consequences approaches does the pain of not doing it become greater than the pain of doing it. The potential pain of fines and late fees becomes a greater pain the closer one gets to April 15th than the pain of taking the time and effort to do the taxes.

Only when the pain of not doing something becomes greater than the pain of doing it will you be motivated to do it. The greater the pain associated with not doing it, the greater the motivation!

In the realm of weight-loss:

When the perceived pain of not losing weight becomes and stays greater than
the perceived pain of the effort to do what it takes to lose weight,
you will be motivated to successfully lose weight and keep it off.

We are motivated by pleasure, but much more so by pain.

Our brains are strongly wired to avoid danger or "pain" to ensure our survival. You'll do a lot more to avoid pain even when there are potentially pleasurable outcomes. For example, people stay stuck in jobs and live lives below what they wish they had, because to them at least it's comfortable and certain. Looking for a better job, going back to school, or starting a small business all involve risk and the potential pain of loss or failure. Despite the potential magnificent pleasure of a better job and a better life, the potential pain of failure or loss associated with going for that pleasure is more motivating. Often times it takes massive pain to motivate people to do things they never thought they could do until they must!
A person gets fired, starts his own small business and now makes 3 times the income and feels real joy in what he does. A person gets a divorce and from her pain reads several books, attends a seminar on relationships, remarries and enjoys a relationship abundantly better than before. A person loses an arm in a car accident, goes into depression and attempts suicide. While recovering he finds his faith, studies, becomes a minister and now 15 years later is pastor of one of the largest churches in the state of Washington.

Behind most personal success stories you'll usually find a painful motivator.

To find your powerful "Whys", ask yourself this question:

**Why do I want to lose weight?**

**Because if I don't, _____will happen**

**Because if I don't, _____could happen**

These reasons must be certain to cause pain or have the real potential to cause massive pain!

## Where Most get Stuck
Most people never really consider WHY they want to lose weight. This is usually taken for granted. To most, it's obvious...who wants to be fat!?! But what most people don't realize is that this generic obvious reason to lose weight doesn't contain nearly enough emotion to blast their willpower to levels needed to forgo delicious high-calorie foods they've been eating for years and to endure the initial pain of starting exercise their body is not accustomed to!

For those that do answer the question of why they want to lose weight, they either draw a blank or can only think of a few "politically correct" reasons like: "*I might get cancer if I don't lose weight*". Health reasons for losing weight are not very motivating because they don't carry much emotional impact until one is actually suffering from a health problem.

There are two ways to find powerful "whys" that will motivate you:

### 1. Associate painful emotions with not changing!

Most people need help digging deep into their self-awareness to find what is most painful for them. For example, a person who finds rejection very painful would be motivated to lose weight if he associated strong feelings of rejection with staying heavy. Find the emotions that you avoid most strongly and associate not changing to those emotions.

Powerfully motivating emotions include:

**rejection**
**loneliness**
**depression**
**humiliation**
**guilt**

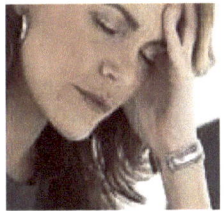

*"If I don't lose weight,*
*how might I experience **rejection** in my life?"*
*"If I don't lose weight,*
*how might I experience **loneliness** in my life?"*
*"If I don't lose weight,*
*how might I experience **guilt** in my life?"*

### 2. Associate losing what is most important to you with not changing.

There's nothing more painful than losing something we love. If I kidnapped your kids, you'd be motivated to do about anything to get them back. Shedding 20 pounds would now suddenly become no problem, just from the single thought that something really bad could happen. In order for the thought of you losing something to motivate you to lose weight, it must be seen as a real possibility. If you thought I was joking, you'd keep eating your 500 calorie bowl of ice cream while watching your favorite TV program at 8pm. The moment you realized I was dead serious, and you perceived the threat of losing your kids as real, you'd be riding the exercise bike at 8 PM with the ice cream in the garbage can!

**"What are the most important things in my life?"**
**"If I don't lose weight, how might I lose or damage these things?"**

## WHY CHANGING WHAT YOU DO IS SO DIFFICULT

Once you've established a powerful "why" or several strong reasons why you *must* lose weight, you'll next need to make some changes to reach your goal. Just like the fly bumping up against the window doing the same thing, you don't want to keep doing the same thing as before, make little progress and end up "dead"! Even when people have a very strong reason why, changing one's habits and routines can be very difficult to overcome in the long run as illustrated by the following story of John:

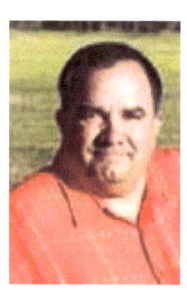

An overweight man named John was told by his doctor that he had a disease that would likely cause his immune system to deteriorate, and eventually shut down in 2-5 years unless he lost 40 pounds and started exercising. Being only 45 and having 2 children - one in 5th grade and one in 7th grade - he definitely had strong reasons to live much longer. So he enthusiastically joined a gym and began to force himself to give up his old eating routine which included, amongst other things, large bowls of ice cream before bed, and junk cereal or cookies with chocolate milk during the night when he'd wake up.

In the first month John lost 13 pounds and was feeling good. The doctor was happy with his progress and encouraged him to keep going. However, results began to slow down and John became frustrated. He found himself skipping workouts and back to his bowls of ice cream and cereal. One bad week turned into a bunch of excuses and self-promises to get back at it at the beginning of the month. He really hated his workouts because he felt embarrassed about how weak and out of shape he was.

After 4 months John regained the 13 pounds he had lost and stopped going to the gym. The arguments at home began to intensify as he was becoming an angry man who believed life had let him down. John began slipping into depression. Despite medication and counseling, John eventually lost his job and sank deeper into despair. Just as the doctor predicted, John died 3 years and 2 months later.

## YOU ARE NOT IN CONTROL OF YOU!

Have you ever been standing in your kitchen and knew you shouldn't open up that bag of nachos in the cupboard, but did anyway. Then after opening the bag, despite knowing you should only have a few chips, ended up eating half the bag! Have you ever woke up in the morning, knew you should go exercise, but decided to stay in your warm bed? You know you should get caught up on the pile of bills that need to be paid, but you decide to watch the game on TV instead?

The first step in successful change is to understand that you are not in charge of you! Meaning, just because you consciously decide to do something, even for a very good reason, you may often FEEL powerfully compelled to do something else, just like John did. Understanding why this happens and how to get control of it is the key to making personal change possible.

**YOU HAVE "2 BRAINS"** Your brain functions in two different ways. I like to think of it as having "2 brains": a conscious brain and a subconscious brain. Your conscious brain is you. It's your active thinking generated by you. Your subconscious brain's main function is the storage of experiences used to create beliefs that help you function in life. For example, if Jill has the experience of getting bit by a dog, she would then believe that dogs are dangerous and she would be more careful around dogs than people who have never been bitten by a dog.

If Jill is bitten again by a dog, her belief that dogs are dangerous would become stronger. If she were bitten a third time by a dog, it might become a conviction to Jill that dogs are vicious and she'd be highly fearful of them and avoiding them would become a "must" for her! If the first experience of getting bitten by the dog was highly traumatic, she could become extremely fearful of dogs with just the single experience because of the high level of emotion. This is how phobias generally occur—a single highly emotional event causes a powerful association of massive pain to that event.

Your beliefs are strengthened by emotion and repetition. Your subconscious is like a powerful computer that guides what you believe and how you feel. Scientists say that every experience you've ever had, good or bad, is stored within your subconscious memory. Through these thousands of filed life experiences (memories), we develop powerful sub-conscious associations like: *"Dogs are vicious!"* or *"Chocolate is to die for!"* Imagine the dilemma Jill would be in if she were invited to a friend's home for chocolate who had a dog! Jill might say over and over to herself and know on a conscious level that not all dogs are vicious, but as soon as she sees the dog, she'd run back to the car with her pulse racing, sweaty palms, and involuntary shaking.

Your subconscious programming associates emotions with things.

Your behavior is controlled by the emotions you experience.

So those who fear dogs could very much consciously want to overcome their fear to be able to visit friends with dogs, but because of their subconscious association, be totally unable to do so. This is the same overlooked problem people face when trying to change eating and exercise habits to lose weight.

People who are overweight have developed strong sub-conscious associations with food that automatically compel them to desire high-calorie foods and dislike low-calorie foods.

People who are overweight have developed strong sub-conscious associations with exercise that automatically compel them to dislike exercise and those people and places associated with it.

Because these subconscious associations are attached strongly to your nervous system, they strongly control your behavior because they make you "feel like" following the conditioned association.

Your brain is constantly making subconscious associations to simplify life. All the things you do "automatically" are subconscious associations your brain has made to make life easier. Imagine if you had to think about what a red traffic light meant, or had to think about how to open an envelope. Learning is the process of your brain making subconscious associations. However, subconscious learned associations can make things in our life become "automatic" when we don't want them to be, as illustrated in the story of Susan:

Susan, an ambitious young attorney, was given a bottle of wine by her boss as a way to thank her for her recent excellent work for the firm. Later that day when she arrived home from work, she decided to open the wine and drink a glass. She felt really good drinking the wine, relaxing and thinking about her accomplishments over the past several months. From this pleasant experience she decides to buy a couple bottles of the same wine to keep at the house to celebrate her future successes.

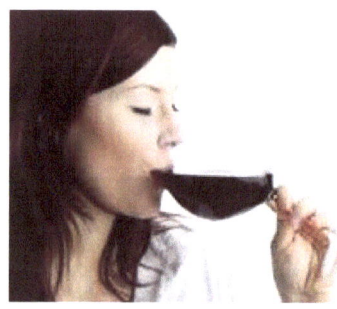

After a few sporadic evenings of enjoying a glass of wine after a hard day at work, over the next six weeks, Susan's subconscious brain begins to associate the emotions of accomplishment and joy with drinking wine after work. Soon she finds herself "feeling like" having a glass of wine every time she gets home from work and her occasional celebration eventually turns into a daily after-work ritual.

Susan didn't consciously set out to drink wine every night. Her subconscious brain simply developed an association between emotions of pleasure and the wine drinking. Because everyone's brain is compelled to do things we associate with emotions of pleasure, Susan is naturally compelled by this invisible force to drink wine after work, enjoy it, and thus keep reinforcing this subconscious association.

After a few months, Susan realizes that drinking wine nightly has been leading her to eat snacks—often half a bag or more of something salty! This has resulted in a 20 pound weight gain which, because she's single, Susan wants to change immediately! So Susan decides consciously to stop her after-work wine drinking and go back to just drinking when she goes to restaurants. The first night after her resolution she returns home and feels the compelling force of her association drawing her to drink a glass of wine and enjoy her normal ritual of sipping a wine while going over the day's events in her head. Consciously she REALLY wants to forgo the wine, but she REALLY "feels" like having a glass of wine! She even hears excuses in her head like: "*I can start this on Monday....it's been a hard week and I deserve to relax.*" This is her subconscious programming trying to avoid the pain of losing the pleasurable emotions it associates with the wine, and now the junk food that always accompanies it.

## SLIP-UPS REINFORCE ASSOCIATIONS

Susan is successful at foregoing wine after work for three weeks, but on the fourth week, she gives in to her desire and has a glass of wine. How Susan thinks about her slip-up is very important to understand. When a person fails at anything, they are faced with two choices:

1. Feel the pain of accepting they screwed up and therefore feel less of themselves.

2. Justify what they did so as to make it not a screw-up.

Because people are motivated away from pain, we're inclined to justify what we did to make it not so bad, or even a good choice. Susan would be naturally drawn to justify her behavior to herself with thoughts like:

- *"I deserve a glass of wine....I can find other ways to lose this weight."*
- *"Wine is good for my health and helps me relax, which makes me a better person."*
- *"I'm a great lawyer; my weight doesn't matter."*

Can you see how these statements would help Susan to feel better about her slip-up? But the danger with these statements is that they all reinforce the association Susan is trying to defeat! The thoughts that she has developed to justify her slip-up now make it much harder to reach her goal of forgoing wine after work. In fact, the slip-up justifying thoughts are typically so powerful, they pull a person back to the behavior for a period of time. Susan might go back to drinking wine for several weeks or months. If she does, she's now reinforced the behavior for several more weeks and her association has become stronger than it was when she first attempted to quit, making breaking it more difficult if she decides to try again. Combine this with her lowered belief in her ability to succeed due to a past failed attempt and we see that Susan would be in a difficult place if she tried to stop her wine drinking again.

Reinforcement of associations, and
a lowered belief in one's ability to succeed,
makes weight-loss for people who have tried and
failed several times nearly impossible!

34

## CHANGE HOW YOU SEE SLIP-UPS

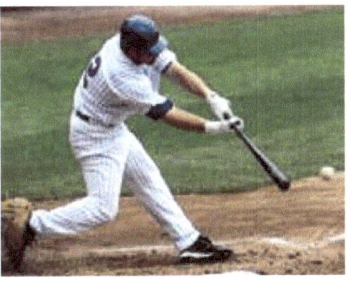

In our natural reaction to feel bad about slip-ups, most people overlook the fact that slip-ups actually help a person become successful. Slip-ups are learning experiences that give you valuable information and insights on what doesn't work, thus getting you closer to what does! This is exactly what a professional baseball player does when he strikes out his first time at bat. Between striking out and his next time at bat, he thinks about what pitches the pitcher threw, what order they came in, and any other distinctions to help him be successful his next time at the plate. Upon going up to bat again, he feels more confident, not less. Even if he strikes out again, the baseball player believes he's made more distinctions and learned more about this pitcher to allow him to smash the ball the next time he's up to bat!

Rather than feeling bad about yourself and automatically inclined to justify yourself, ask: *"What can I learn from this?"* Get curious and excited because the answers to this question will get you closer to your goal! Had Susan asked herself this question, she may have learned the reason for her slip-up that day was because an unusually stressful day at the office broke her motivation to forgo the attractive de-stressing power of a glass of wine. A solution that could come from this knowledge might be next time she has a stressful day at work, to instead go directly to the gym to work off the stress before going home.

Slip-ups provide you with
valuable information needed
to make the changes to your approach
necessary for success!

# WHY WILLPOWER IS NOT VERY POWERFUL

If not indulged, an association, like a memory, will weaken over time. How long this will take depends on how strongly the association is recorded into the subconscious. The strength of an association is determined by how many times it has been repeated or experienced and how emotional each experience is.

### Strength of an Association =
(1st experience x emotional strength) +
(2nd experience x emotional strength) +
(3rd experience x emotional strength) +
(4th experience x emotional strength) +
(5th experience x emotional strength) + ...

In the case of Susan's after work wine drinking association, the number of times she drank wine after work, and how pleasurable each time was to her, determines how strong her association is. From the above formula, you can see that something experienced just a few times but in which each event was highly emotional can develop an equal or stronger association than something experienced several times with less emotional impact.

## EMOTIONS, NOT INTENTIONS, MOTIVATE YOU
Human beings are motivated and compelled by our emotions. When you feel angry, do you do things differently
than when you feel sad? When you feel joyful, do you communicate differently than when you feel rejected? You had planned to clean the basement today, but instead found yourself watching TV and eating cookies because you felt overwhelmed and hurt by something your spouse said this

morning. Your feelings control what you do far more than what you'd like to do consciously.

Using willpower to stop doing something you feel compelled to do, like smoke, overeat or skip exercise is the process of ignoring the powerful force of your emotions (feelings) associated with that particular something you are trying to change.

If you are using willpower to quit smoking, you are *trying to ignore* the pleasurable feelings you currently associate with smoking.

If you are using willpower to not eat treats at night before bed, you are *trying to ignore* the pleasurable feelings you currently associate with eating treats in the evening.

If you are using willpower to get to the gym to exercise, you are *trying to ignore* the negative feelings you currently associate with exercising at the gym.

Ignoring your feelings is very difficult. Think of your feelings as an alarm going off. Alarms are difficult to ignore. How long does the **beep, beep, beep, beep, beep, beep** have to go on before you give into the alarm and go turn it off? Think of your associations the same way. When you feel the desire to eat cookies at night, your cookie association starts to **beep, beep, beep, beep, beep** in your head until you go to the kitchen and get some cookies! Can you ignore this alarm? It can be done, but it's very difficult. Why? Because the human brain can't NOT think

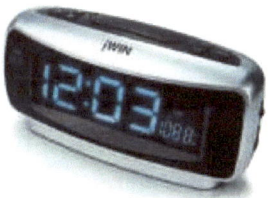

about something. Right now, try to not think about a yellow school bus. Whatever you do DON'T think about or visualize a yellow school bus. You can think about anything else, but not a yellow school bus. What is happening? You're thinking about a yellow school bus! In fact, the more you try NOT to think about it, the more you do! But if I called you on the phone and told you about something hilarious that happened to me today, your thinking focus would shift from the yellow school bus to my story.

Trying not to think about something<br>makes you think about it even more.

The alarm does eventually go off. Perhaps you go and brush your teeth and minty taste of the toothpaste signals your brain that it's time for bed which causes the cookie alarm to go off. Or you start reading a book or a newspaper article and your mind's focus moves to what you're reading and the alarm goes off. Each time the cookie alarm is ignored, it weakens. So over time the **beep, beep, beep** becomes **beep, beep,** beep, beep. However, this could be over a period of many months before the "*beep*" becomes weak enough to no longer strongly compel you.

Willpower works better for things you can completely eliminate and live without like smoking or wine. If a smoker decides to quit, each day he goes without smoking, the subconscious association weakens. When it comes to controlling what you eat, because it's impossible to completely eliminate pleasure foods from your life, the associations are constantly being reinforced making willpower less effective. For example, let's say you have an association with ice cream in the evening after dinner. For three months you forgo ice cream and you feel the pull to have a bowl has weakened significantly, but it's still there and you still need to use willpower to not go to the basement freezer. Then you have a birthday party and eat cake and ice cream or you decide to have an ice cream cone with your kids. Because you haven't had ice cream in three months the ice cream tastes awesome, unbelievable, amazing! Your brain gets hit with an experience associating MASSIVE PLEASURE = ICE CREAM! So the association you used willpower to weaken just got a supercharged re-association, putting you back closer to where you started.

## WHY NOT JUST CHANGE THE ASSOCIATION?

Once a person understands how learned subconscious associations control what one "feels like" doing, a bulb lights up in most people's heads. One realizes that it would be easier to get rid of or change the association and be free from its strong "invisible" pull toward the behavior we want so badly to change. But because understanding the subconscious brain is new to most people, they assume they wouldn't have a clue how to do this. But actually, everyone has done it!

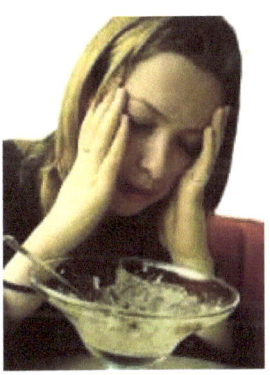

If you have ever been really sick from eating a certain food you used to love, and after the painful experience found that food totally unattractive, you successfully changed a subconscious association. Have you ever had a big fight or had a very bad experience in what used to be your favorite restaurant, and now you never go there because the thought of going there makes you feel that same painful emotion from the memory of what happened?

Changing an association is not rocket science—actually it's brain science. To free yourself from the strong invisible pull of an association, you simply create a highly emotional experience that overpowers and collapses the old association.

In Susan's case, she would create a highly emotional experience that attached pain (or the loss of pleasure) to drinking wine after work. To collapse an association, you associate an opposite emotion until its strength is greater than the old association. The strength of the opposite association depends on the number of opposite experiences and the emotional intensity of each experience.

(1st opposite experience x emotional strength) +
(2nd opposite experience x emotional strength) +
(3rd opposite experience x emotional strength) +
(4th opposite experience x emotional strength) +
(5th opposite experience x emotional strength) + ...

*must become GREATER than the current association.*

## REAL EXPERIENCES VS. POTENTIAL CONSEQUENCES

The problem with breaking an association lies in the fact that the associations we want to break have been reinforced by real experiences. Each time Susan drank the wine, she felt the pleasurable emotions of accomplishment and joy. Each time Jill got bit by a dog, she experienced the painful emotions of fear and physical pain. Real opposite experiences would be if Susan got massively sick from drinking wine or Jill had several experiences with loving dogs. But the problem is that Jill would never get near any dog, and Susan might go through a lot of wine before ever getting sick! So when going about the business of purposefully changing your associations, the only tools to use are the potential consequences of continuing the behavior.

*One must create potential consequences which seem so negative that continuing the behavior is no longer worth the pleasure gained.*

Awareness of the potential negative consequences is the first step. Human beings easily ignore or don't even consider the many possible consequences when we get focused on fulfilling an emotional need. The second step is to take all those potential consequences and greatly ramp-up their emotional impact so as to massively increase the desire to avoid them!

## RAMP UP & MAGNIFY THE EMOTIONAL IMPACT

If I were to suggest to Susan a consequence of her continued wine drinking could be a permanent weight gain of 20 pounds, resulting in living single for much longer than she wanted, it would have some emotional impact on her.

However, if I were to have her visualize a scenario of being harshly rejected by a man she was very attracted to, the experience of such a consequence would have the more powerful emotional impact needed to change her association!

**Susan's Current Association**

Accomplishment and joy with drinking wine

**New Association**

Rejection from weight gain from drinking wine

For most people, the thought of themselves using visualization to create emotional experiences seems like a foreign language, but in actuality we do it every day! Anything that happened or could happen that we think about is a process of visualization. If it's not happening in the present, then you must be visualizing something that happened in the past or could happen in the future. Most people are really good at visualizing negative things—that's our natural wiring to avoid pain and discomfort. When you feel worried, you are visualizing a future outcome that you believe could go bad. When you feel overwhelmed and sick to your stomach, you're visualizing the potential negative outcomes of not getting everything done.

I have a friend who heard from someone that her ex-husband was going to drain their bank account before their divorce was final. She was worried sick that she'd lose all the savings she worked so hard to accumulate. I told her that she's immobilizing herself over something that *might* happen. But my words didn't help her much, because she could vividly "see" her ex-husband going down to the bank and closing the account. Her visualization of this possible event was deeply emotional to her! She later found out he was just "talking big" to a friend, just like I thought.

Kids are really good using their imagination to picture things that are not real. They visualize the color, shape and size of the monster in the closet and to them it seems so real and scary. They visualize an imaginary friend they are reading to or playing with. The cool thing about visualization is that your subconscious brain does not distinguish between a real experience and an imagined experience that seems real. Ever watch a scary movie and go lock your doors? You're visualizing. Ever wake-up from a dream and think it was real for a few minutes until you realize you were just dreaming (visualizing)? The neurological pathways of a visualized experience and a real experience are the same. This has been proven in many studies, one of which involved basketball players visualizing shooting successful free throws. The group that visualized successful free throws had higher improvements in shooting free throws than the group that actually shot them!

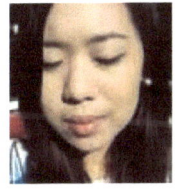

The greater the emotions you feel during the visualization, the more you'll want to avoid experiencing the potential consequences of your current behavior.

Perhaps the best description of this force on one's behavior is what happened to Ebenezer Scrooge in the movie "*A Christmas Carol*". Old Ebenezer was visited by three ghosts who showed him the immensely painful future consequences of his current behaviors. If the ghosts had just sat Ebenezer down and described to him what could happen if he kept up his old ways, it would have done little to nothing to motivate him to change. When Ebenezer "sees" and "hears" what painful things could happen, the emotional impact is strong enough to change even a man as set in his ways as Ebenezer Scrooge!

## ROLE MODELS CAN CHANGE ASSOCIATIONS WITHOUT TRYING

People are highly influenced by others, especially friends, co-workers, and family. We are drawn to those like ourselves and want to "fit in" and be approved of by those around us. The people we admire are especially influential in our lives. By just being around a person you'd like to be like, you'll be automatically drawn to take on their beliefs, and dispose of your old beliefs that contradict theirs. This can occur indirectly when you read about or watch videos of people you'd like to be like. This natural role model affect is most potent when you get around a live person. For the goal of weight-loss, this means hiring a personal trainer or weight-loss coach to be your role model.

The key is to find a trainer/coach you highly admire. The more you admire them, the more you'll be drawn to adopt their beliefs (associations). When they talk about what they eat, when they go to bed, when they exercise, how they live their life, you are compelled to do the same because you want to be like them!

What makes a person admirable and a great role model? There are many characteristics, but when it comes down to what gives someone great role model power, it all boils down to three key traits:

- Confidence
- Attitude
- Trustworthiness

When they say "opposites attract" it means human beings

are naturally drawn to people who have the traits they don't have or wish they had more of. Most people, especially those that are struggling with their weight, lack a strong inner confidence and are thus naturally attracted to those who have high levels of genuine confidence. You know the people that walk into a room who are just glowing with confidence in the way they walk, talk, hold their body, make eye contact easily and seem so at ease with themselves. This has nothing to do with their physical attractiveness, but it's an inner energy that is impossible to overlook, and I believe is one of the most powerful forces on the planet. Confident people are usually physically attractive as well because they have high levels of healthy self-love which makes taking care of themselves a high priority. We all wish we were more confident, so when we meet someone who's got it in large quantities we are naturally attracted to them. Attractive and confident people are like personal change magnets. They just pull you in!

The second trait of an effective role model is their positive attitude. These people live life with high levels of happiness and gratitude. Even though on the surface these people might make us mad or drive us crazy, deep inside we wish we felt the same way. Most people don't feel happy or grateful on a regular basis because we live with the belief that if we had fewer problems, had more stuff and accomplished more things, we'd be happier. So when we see happy, grateful people, we think subconsciously they must be following some success formula, allowing them to have fewer problems, have more stuff and accomplish more! We're naturally drawn to want to have that same success formula too!

The third trait of an effective role model is trustworthiness. These people give you a feeling deep inside that you can 100% believe & trust them. It comes mostly from how "genuine" and "real" the person seems to you. A trustworthy person demonstrates total congruence between what they say and do. Through their body language you can tell this person is someone you can believe and through a feeling of rapport with the person, which comes from the feeling that this person understands you and cares about you, you know you can trust them.

If Susan were to hire a personal trainer she highly admired who believed that wine and alcohol just leads to big problems and makes people fat, she would be quite compelled to stop drinking wine because she would now associate drinking with the painful emotion of rejection from a person from whom she strongly seeks approval! Changing becomes nearly automatic if the role model's level of influence through your admiration is very high.

Role Model Power (Influence) =
The Level of Regard (Admiration)

High-Power Role Models:
- Parents to their Children
- Popular Classmates, Entertainment and Sports Icons to Teenagers
- Older Siblings to younger Siblings
- Close Friends
- Confident & Positive Personal Trainer to Client

## HOW CAN ANYONE LIKE BEER?

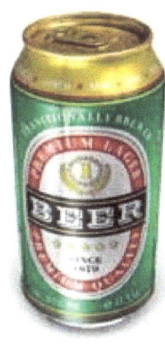 Why most people are compelled to try a naturally unpleasant tasting beverage like beer, is a good example of how role models can influence a person's associations. I remember the first time I tried a beer. I must have been about 10 or 11 when I snuck a can from my Grandpa's (role model) barn refrigerator where he had his stash of Pabst Blue Ribbon. I remember how bitter and strong it tasted and how repulsed I was, thinking "*How could anybody stand this stuff?*" Pop or Kool-Aid seemed infinitely more appealing.

Things changed when I hit my senior year in high school and then college. Older popular classmates (role models) were drinking and the parties I wanted to be a part of involved everyone drinking beer. I began to associate strong feelings of fitting in, getting girls and becoming an adult with drinking beer. Add in the benefit of alcohol reducing my insecurities, making me feel more confident, and you can easily see why I and most insecure young adults decide to drink beer despite its naturally foul taste.

As my taste buds and nose were experiencing the taste and smell of beer, my brain was experiencing strong and highly appealing thoughts of fitting in, being popular and getting girls! With just a few cans of Milwaukee's finest, my brain taught my tongue and nose to "like" the taste of beer! This proves, by the way, that "taste" is not a genetic or random personal preference, but actually a neurological association that can be changed. Yes, you can teach your brain to love and want the foods you currently don't "like".

**SUMMARY** I hope this book has given you several "a-ha" moments, and most of all helped you understand what I meant by weight- loss failure is NOT your fault! There's a typical path that most people follow when they decide to make a personal change like weight-loss. This is the path of using willpower to overcome one's natural desires. Statistics show that more than 90% of people who take this path end up failing in the long-run.

A better path is the one in which you remove the invisible barriers that powerfully pull you back to old behaviors. This allows for the behaviors you WANT to be reinforced without the old habits constantly popping up and destroying your progress and causing you to fail.

## WHICH WAY ARE YOU HEADING?

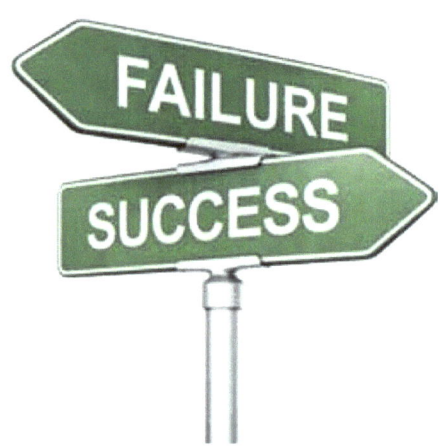

# Typical Path of Failure

1. Decide to change
2. Force new behaviors with willpower
3. Constant battle between what you feel like doing and your will
4. Slip-ups seen as failures of one's will/ability
5. Slip-ups reinforce old associations
6. Go back to old behaviors

# New Path for Success!

1. Decide to change
2. Find & create motivating reasons for change
3. Learn how to control emotions & states
4. Change the associations of the behaviors you want to change
   a) Get a role model
   b) Self-reprogramming
5. Your will and what you feel like doing grow more similar
5. Slip-ups are seen as natural in the change process
7. Slip-ups help reinforce new associations
8. New behaviors become what you feel like doing

# WHAT DO I DO NOW?

## Step 1: Get role models into your life.

I can't emphasize this enough. Getting other human beings into your life that have rejected the associations you are trying to reject and are living the associations you are trying to develop is tremendously powerful! It's SO powerful, it can get a teenager whose taste buds are hooked on sweet beverages to try and develop a liking for bitter-tasting beer!

If the only people in your life are those who share the associations you are trying to change, they will keep reinforcing what you're trying to change and this uphill battle will quickly extinguish your resolve and crush your willpower. This is THE core reason so many fail at weight-loss.

The best place to find people who are living with the associations you want to develop is at a gym! That's the REAL value of a membership at a Fitness Center - the opportunity to be around influential role models of all shapes, sizes and ages! Sure, a variety of equipment is an asset to keep up an exercise program, but if you don't adopt an inner desire to work out, you won't use any of the equipment!

One of the biggest mistakes people make when attempting to lose weight is to avoid others who are what they'd like to be. They think, "*I don't want to join a gym and be around all those fit & healthy people...I'd feel like a schmuck!*" So instead they spend money on home exercise equipment and videos and think they will be successful in their own little private bubble.

Fear is the controlling force that drives people away from taking successful action; specifically the fear of embarrassment or disapproval from others. But these fears are really not true. Most people in gyms are just like you and those in great shape remember how they felt years ago and as such welcome new folks who want to make a positive change. As a gym owner, I know this to be a fact. The fit people you see in the gym LOVE to help beginners because exercise and eating healthy for a purpose is our passion!

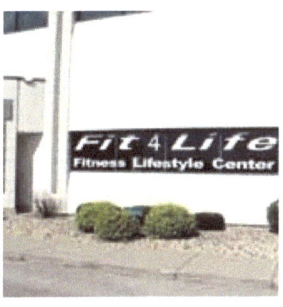

The truth is that the fit people in the gym are really waiting for you to ask: *"excuse me, you look very experienced. I'm new here and would you have a second to show me how to use this machine correctly?"* With that single sincere request by you, a new friendship could be born with a person who could become your "gym friend" and your role model to automatically pull you to the inner changes you could never make isolated at home on your own!

### Step 2: Hire a personal role model (trainer).
The value of hiring a trainer is not in the amount of knowledge they have about exercise and weight loss. In fact, I truly believe a trainer can have too much knowledge and overwhelm their clients. Look for a trainer who not only will teach you the skills of how to exercise and eat for the results you want, but most importantly will share their thoughts, attitudes and beliefs with you.

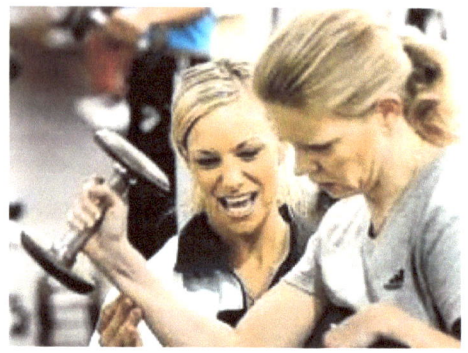

Look for a trainer who you feel attracted to by their personality. They don't necessarily need to be your same age or sex, but you need to be very compelled by them. Remember a role model's power comes from how much you admire their confidence and attitude, and how much trust you feel with that person. Look to hire a trainer that you hear a voice inside you say: *"Wow, I want to be like him (her)!"* It's a good idea to visit with more than one trainer until you find the one that you feel has role model power for you...it's that important!

A great coach understands that you have to feel good to be able to do the things consistently that causes weight-loss and will teach you skills and give you tools to manage and eliminate the stress and negative feelings in your life that hold you back.

A great coach will sit down with you and go over why you want to lose weight. He or she will help you find your powerful "whys" that make changing a "must" instead of a "should".

A great coach will help you identify the inner associations you have about food and exercise, and help you destroy them by associating massive pain to keeping them, and massive pleasure to adopting new associations.

Unfortunately, finding a true "Coach" might be difficult. Most gyms have helpful and caring trainers who would love to help you start and implement an exercise and eating program, but know very little about what I just described and what you read about in this book. Because of this you should…

**Step 3: Let me be your Coach & Role model**! If you want to implement what's in this book, what better person to teach you than the author!

Go to my program www.newbodychoice.net

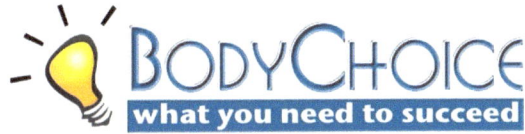

Or my Defeat Craving program at: www.defeatcravings.com

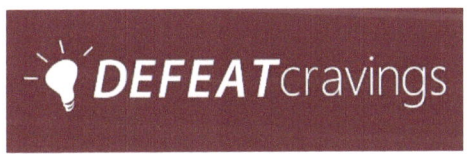

*All the Best,*
*Talk to you*
*soon!*

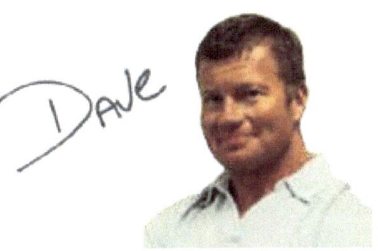

**N**OTES: